HEALTH TECH BOOK SERIES

DO NOT BE AFRAID OF SWINE FLU

FAST SOLUTION IS AVAILABLE IN YOUR KITCHEN

BY

Professor Awad Mansour

Professor of Chemical & Pharmaceutical Engineering

Formerly with University of Akron

Ohio U.S.A

First Edition
2009

HEALTH TECH BOOK SERIES

Published by Health Tech Technologies Ltd. 2009

Copyright @2009 Professor Awad Mansour

First printing 2009

Mansour, Awad

DO NOT BE AFRAID OF SWINE FLUE

/Awad Mansour—1st ed.2009.

124 p.

ISBN:1-4392-4941-5

EAN: 9781439249413

1. Swine Flu 2.Natural Remedies   I. Title

Printed in the United States of America

Table of Contents

Acknowledgment

The effort of reviewing this book by Prof. Dr. Fayez Khasawna, the former President of Yarmouk University is highly appreciated.

INTRODUCTION

Dr.Mercola wrote(www.mercola.com):
From: Associated Press, April 27, 2009,
http://www.google.com/hostednews/ap/article/ALeqM5hceWV2_C
u7yoSvw9iNYZ90-qnCyQD97R2FVG3

Your Fear Will Make Some People VERY Rich in Today's Crumbling Economy

Tamiflu (oseltamivir phosphate) is approved for treatment of uncomplicated influenza A and B in children 1 year of age or older. It is also approved for prevention of influenza in people 13 years or older. It's part of a group of anti-influenza drugs called neuraminidase inhibitors, which work by blocking a viral enzyme that helps the influenza virus to invade cells in your respiratory tract. According to the Associated Press *at least one financial analyst estimates up to $388 million worth of Tamiflu sales in the near future[10] -- and that's without a pandemic outbreak. More than half a dozen pharmaceutical companies, including Gilead Sciences Inc., Roche, GlaxoSmithKline and other companies with a stake in flu treatments and detection, have seen a rise in their shares in a matter of days, and will likely see revenue boosts if the swine flu outbreak continues to spread.*

Swine flue is extremely convenient for governments that would have very soon have to dispose of billions of dollars of Tamiflu stock, which they bought to counter avian flu, or H5N1. The US government ordered 20 million doses, costing $2 billion, in October, 2005, and around that time the UK government ordered 14.6 million doses. Tamiflu's manufacturer, Roche, has confirmed that the shelf life of its anti-viral is three years.

As soon as Homeland Security declared a health emergency, 25 percent -- about 12 million doses -- of Tamiflu and Relenza treatment courses were released from the nation's stockpile. However, beware that the declaration also allows unapproved tests and drugs to be administered to children. Many health- and government officials are more than willing to take that chance with your life, and the life of your child. But are you?

Tamiflu Loaded With Side Effects, Including Death and Can Only Reduce Symptoms by 36 Hours at BEST

Please realize that Tamiflu is NOT a safe drug Serious side effects include convulsions, delirium or delusions, and <u>14 deaths in children </u>and teens as a result of neuropsychiatric problems and brain infections Japan actually banned Tamiflu for children in 2007.

Remember, Tamiflu went through some rough times not too long ago, as the dangers of this drug came to light when, in 2007, the <u>FDA finally began investigating some 1,800 adverse event reports related to the drug</u>.

Additionally common side effects of Tamiflu include:Nausea ,Vomiting,Diarrhea,Headache Dizziness,Fatigue,Cough

All in all, the very symptoms you're trying to avoid. Additionally, Tamiflu has been reported to be ineffective against seasonal flu outbreaks, and may not be sufficient to combat an epidemic or pandemic.

But making matters worse, some patients with influenza are at HIGHER risk for secondary bacterial infections when on Tamiflu. And secondary bacterial infections, as I mentioned earlier, was likely the REAL cause of the mass fatalities during the 1918 pandemic!

But here's the real kicker. When Tamiflu is used as directed (twice daily for 5 days) it can ONLY reduce the duration of your influenza symptoms by 1 to 1 ½ days, according to the official data.

Why on earth would anyone want to take a drug that has a chance of killing you, was banned in Japan, is loaded with side effects that mimic the flu itself, costs over $100, and AT BEST can only provide 36 hours of SYMPTOM relief. Just doesn't make any sense.

Please recognize that there is serious revenue in Tamiflu. The Financial Times reports that governments around the world have previously stockpiled 220 million doses in preparation for a pandemic that has yet to appear. The cost of this preparation is $7 billion dollars.

In this book the reader will discover that swine flu is a week virus and can be avoided by simple natural and effective 100% safe means(secret means are discussed in details in Chapter 10 of this book) and the reader will discover that there is no justifications for his/her fear!!!

CHAPTER I

What Is Swine Flu?

What is Swine Flu?

From **Wikipedia**, the free encyclopedia & **CDC** (Centers for Disease Control and Prevention):

Swine influenza (also called **swine flu, hog flu and pig flu**) is a respiratory disease which infects pigs caused by influenza type A virus.There are regular outbreaks among herds of pigs, where the disease causes high levels of illness but is rarely fatal

It tends to spread in autumn and winter but can circulate all year round.There are many different types of swine flu and, like human flu, the infection is constantly changing.

Swine flu does not normally infect humans, although sporadic **cases do occur usually in people who have had close contact with pigs.**

There have also been rare documented cases of humans passing the infection to other humans.

Human to human transmission of swine flu is thought to spread in the same way as seasonal flu – through coughing and sneezing.

The outbreak in Mexico seems to involve a new type of swine flu that contains DNA that is typically found in avian(bird flu virus H5N1) and human ordinary viruses.

The World Health Organization has confirmed at least some of the cases are caused by this new strain of H1N1

"We are very, very concerned," World Health Organization

(WHO) spokesman Thomas Abraham said. "We have what appears to be a novel virus and it has spread from human to human"

It is genetically different from the fully human H1N1 seasonal influenza virus that has been circulating globally for the past few years. It contains DNA that is typical to avian, swine and human viruses, including elements from European and Asian swine viruses.

When any new strain of flu emerges that acquires the ability to pass from person to person, it is monitored very closely in case it has the potential to spark a pandemic

The WHO has changed the threat level warning for a pandemic.

H1N1 is different from other strains of influenza. This particular strain of influenza has not been previously exposed to humans before, so there are no built up immunities to it. This is what makes it so serious. At the current time there is no preventative drug that you can take in order to avoid getting it. That is why people who are elderly, very young or those who have compromised immune systems must be extremely careful to avoid getting the flu.

It was renamed H1N1 influenza A to avoid people making a connection to pigs. This is similar in some ways to the flu that hit the world decades ago. However it is proving to be more serious. The outbreak is becoming serious because nobody has any immunity to this particular strain of influenza. It is estimated that approximately 1 in 4 people who come into contact with swine flu will contract it.

Dr Michael Osterholm, a public health expert at the University of Minnesota, said given how quickly flu can spread around the globe, if these are the first signs of a pandemic, then there are probably cases incubating in other parts of the world already

There is no vaccine that specifically protects against swine flu, and it was unclear how much protection current human flu vaccines might offer!!!

Scientists have long been concerned that a new flu virus could launch a worldwide pandemic of a killer disease.

A new pandemic flu virus could evolve when different flu viruses infect a pig, a person or a bird, mingling their genetic material. The resulting hybrid could spread quickly because people would have no natural immunity against it.

The most notorious flu pandemic is thought to have killed at least 40 million people worldwide in 1918-19. Two other, less deadly flu pandemics struck in 1957 and 1968

Electron microscope image of the re-assorted H1N1 influenza virus photographed at the CDC Influenza Laboratory. The viruses are 80–120 nanometres in diameter(nanometer means 1 billionth of a meter).

A **S**wine **I**nfluenza **V**irus (**SIV**) is any strain of the influenza family of viruses that is usually hosted by pigs. As of 2009, the known SIV strains are the influenza C virus and the subtypes of the influenza A virus known as H1N1, H1N2, H3N1, H3N2, and

H2N3. Swine flu is common throughout pig populations worldwide.

People who work with pigs, especially people with intense exposures, are at increased risk of catching swine flu. Approximately 1% to 4% of pigs that get swine flu die from it. It is spread among pigs by direct and indirect contact, aerosols, and from pigs that are infected but do not have symptoms. In the mid-20th century, identification of influenza subtypes became possible, which allows accurate diagnosis of transmission to humans. In humans, the symptoms of swine flu are similar to those of flu and of flu-like illness in general, namely chills, fever, sore throat, muscle pains, severe headache, coughing, weakness and general discomfort. **Pigs can also become infected with human influenza, and this appears to have happened during the 1918 flu pandemic.**

The 2009 swine flu outbreak in humans is due to a new strain of influenza A virus subtype H1N1 that contains genes closely related to swine influenza. The origin of this new strain is unknown. However, the World Organization for Animal Health (OIE) reports that this strain has not been isolated in pigs. This strain can be transmitted from human to human, and causes the normal symptoms of influenza.

Classification of Influenza Types

- Of the three strains of influenza viruses that cause human flu, two also cause influenza in pigs, with Influenza virus A being common in pigs and Influenza virus C being rare. Influenza virus B has not been reported in pigs. Within Influenza virus A and Influenza virus C, the strains found in pigs and humans are largely distinct, although due to re-assortment there have been transfers of genes among strains crossing swine, bird, and human species boundaries.

Influenza C

Influenza C viruses infect both humans and pigs, but do not infect birds.

Transmission between pigs and humans have occurred in the past. For example, influenza C caused small outbreaks of a mild form of flu amongst children in Japan and California. Due to its limited host range and the lack of genetic diversity in influenza C, this form of influenza does not cause pandemics in humans.

Influenza A

Swine influenza is known to be caused by influenza A subtypes H1N1, H1N2,H3N1 H3N2, and H2N3 In pigs, three influenza A virus subtypes (H1N1, H3N2, and H1N2) are the most common strains worldwide. In the United States, the H1N1 subtype was exclusively prevalent among swine populations before 1998. However, since late August 1998, H3N2 subtypes have been isolated from pigs. As of 2004, H3N2 virus isolates in US swine and turkey stocks were triple re-assortants, containing genes from human (HA, NA, and PB1), swine (NS, NP, and M), and avian (PB2 and PA) lineages.

Novel H1N1 Flu in Humans

Are there human infections with novel H1N1 virus in the U.S.?

CDC has determined that novel H1N1 virus is contagious and is spreading from human to human. However, at this time, it is not known how easily the virus spreads between people.

How severe is illness associated with novel H1N1 flu virus?

It is not known at this time how severe novel H1N1 flu virus will be in the general population. **In seasonal flu, there are certain people that are at higher risk of serious flu-related complications**. This includes people 65 years and older, children younger than five years old, pregnant women, and people of any age with certain chronic medical conditions. Early indications are that pregnancy and other previously recognized medical conditions that increase the risk of influenza-related complications, like asthma and diabetes, also appear to be associated with increased risk of complications from novel H1N1 virus infection as well.

One thing that appears to be different from seasonal influenza is that adults older than 64 years do not yet appear to be at increased risk of novel H1N1-related complications thus far in the outbreak. CDC is conducting laboratory studies to see if certain people might have natural immunity to this virus, depending on their age. Early reports indicate that no children and few adults younger than 60 years old have existing antibody to novel H1N1 flu virus; however, about one-third of adults older than 60 may have antibodies against this virus. It is unknown how much, if any, protection may be afforded against novel H1N1 flu by any existing antibody

How does novel H1N1 flu compare to seasonal flu in terms of its severity and infection rates?

CDC is still learning about the severity of novel H1N1 flu virus. At this time, there is not enough information to predict how severe novel H1N1 flu outbreak will be in terms of illness and death or how it will compare with seasonal influenza

With seasonal flu, we know that seasons vary in terms of timing, duration and severity. **Seasonal influenza can cause mild to severe illness, and at times can lead to death. Each year, in the United States, on average 36,000 people die from flu-related complications and more than 200,000 people are hospitalized from flu-related causes**. Of those hospitalized, 20,000 are children younger than 5 years old. Over 90% of deaths and about 60 percent of hospitalization occur in people older than 65.

So far, with novel H1N1 flu, the largest number of novel H1N1 flu confirmed and probable cases have occurred in people between the ages of 5 and 24-years-old. At this time, there are few cases and no deaths reported in people older than 64 years old, which is unusual when compared with seasonal flu. However, pregnancy and other previously recognized high risk medical conditions from seasonal influenza appear to be associated with increased risk of complications from this novel H1N1

How does novel H1N1 virus spread?

Spread of novel H1N1 virus is thought to be happening in the same way that seasonal flu spreads. Flu viruses are spread mainly from person to person through coughing or sneezing by people with influenza. Sometimes people may become infected by touching something with flu viruses on it and then touching their mouth or nose.

How long can an infected person spread this virus to others?

At the current time, CDC believes that this virus has the same properties in terms of spread as seasonal flu viruses. With seasonal flu, studies have shown that people may be contagious from one day before they develop symptoms to up to 7 days after they get sick. Children, especially younger children, might potentially be contagious for longer periods. CDC is studying the virus and its capabilities to try to learn more and will provide more information as it becomes available.

Exposure is not thought to spread novel H1N1 Flu

Is there a risk from drinking water?

Tap water that has been treated by conventional disinfection processes does not likely pose a risk for transmission of influenza viruses. Current drinking water treatment regulations provide a high degree of protection from viruses. No research has been completed on the susceptibility of novel H1N1 flu virus to conventional drinking water treatment processes. However, recent studies have demonstrated that free chlorine levels typically used in drinking water treatment are adequate to inactivate highly pathogenic H5N1 avian influenza. It is likely that other influenza viruses such as novel H1N1 would also be similarly inactivated by chlorination. To date, there have been no documented human cases of influenza caused by exposure to influenza-contaminated drinking water.

Can novel H1N1 flu virus be spread through water in swimming pools, spas, water parks, interactive fountains, and other treated recreational water venues?

Influenza viruses infect the human upper respiratory tract. There has never been a documented case of influenza virus infection associated with water exposure. Recreational water that has been treated at CDC recommended disinfectant levels does not likely pose a risk for transmission of influenza viruses. No research has been completed on the susceptibility of novel H1N1 influenza virus to chlorine and other disinfectants used in swimming pools, spas, water parks, interactive fountains, and other treated recreational venues. However, recent studies have demonstrated that free chlorine levels recommended by CDC (1–3 parts per million [ppm or mg/L] for pools and 2–5 ppm for spas) are adequate to disinfect avian influenza A (H5N1) virus. It is likely that other influenza viruses such as novel H1N1 virus would also be similarly disinfected by chlorine.

Can novel H1N1 flu virus be spread at recreational water venues outside of the water?

Yes, recreational water venues are no different than any other group setting. The spread of this novel H1N1 flu is thought to be happening in the same way that seasonal flu spreads. Flu viruses are spread mainly from person to person through coughing or sneezing of people with influenza. Sometimes people may become infected by touching something with flu viruses on it and then touching their mouth or nose

Why have we stopped calling it SWINE FLU?

The name was changed to dispel the misconception that the virus is derived from pig products.

The name change came after about 15 countries, including China and Russia, slapped restrictions on imports of live pigs and pork from the United States, Canada and Mexico, and after Egypt needlessly ordered that all 250,000 pigs in the country be killed.

The CDC was the first to use the term "swine flu" after initial analysis showed the nature of the virus.

Further tests revealed it also contained genetic material from a human flu virus and avian flu virus. After undergoing genetic changes (called "antigenic shift"), what likely started as a swine flu has now become a human- swine flu.

Aren't pigs now getting this flu?

The Canadian Food Inspection Agency reports that a herd of pigs in Alberta tested positive for this H1N1 strain. The pigs were likely exposed to the virus from a hog farm worker who had recently returned from Mexico and had been exhibiting flu-like symptoms

The pigs then developed the symptoms of flu: a sudden fever, a barking cough, sneezing and decreased appetite. All the infected pigs have recovered, as has the individual who travelled to Mexico.

How did this new strain develop?

No body knows till this moment.

It is likely that pigs were the "reservoir"or "**incubator**" where the virus developed, since pigs are notorious "mixing bowls" for viruses. Onething we are certain of: this new strain of flu contains some elements of swine influenza virus.

The investigation on how did it develop could take a while and it's possible the answer will never be found.

Why is a new flu strain worrisome?

If an influenza virus changes and becomes a new strain against which people have little or no immunity -- and if this new strain can easily spread from person to person and cause severe illness in a high percentage of people that it infects -- the seeds would be sown for a pandemic that could sicken and kill many people around the world.

Though epidemiologists have been warning for years that it's just a matter of time before a new strain of the flu emerges that has the potential to kill millions **Professor Mansour in the following chapters of this book shows millions of people all over the world that THERE IS NO PLACE FOR FEAR OF SWINE FLU, AND, THAT IT CAN BE TREATED MUCH EASIER THAN ORDINARY FLU IN ONE DAY ONLY!!**

What is a pandemic?

A pandemic is an epidemic of infectious disease that has spread across a large region, such as across continents or worldwide. But a pandemic can be mild or severe, depending on how many deaths the disease causes

When most of us think of flu pandemics, we think of the 1918 Spanish Flu. But remember that the 1968 Hong Kong flu epidemic killed only about 700,000 worldwide. That's less than many yearly outbreaks of garden-variety seasonal flu

If the current human swine flu outbreak is declared a pandemic, it is more likely to be of the 1968 variety because we have been exposed to several parts of this virus before. We also have good public health systems that are ready for a pandemic with antiviral medications and infection control measures. **BESIDES, WE HAVE A NEW SERIES OF ALTERNATIVE NATURAL ANTI-VIRAL**

AND ANTI-BACTERIAL MEANS TO PROTECT OURSELVES AVAILABLE IN HEALTH STORES AND IN OUR KITCHINS!!!!!

As well, the number of deaths among the people contacting the disease from this virus has been relatively low. Outside of Mexico, there has been only few death cases. In other countries, such as Canada, it's causing such mild illness that it's running its course in two to three days, in some cases without any treatment!!!

How is the virus transmitted?

From contact with infected pigs.

From human-to-human swine flu is believed to occur the same way as seasonal flu, mainly through coughing or sneezing of people infected with the influenza virus.

People also can become infected by touching something with flu viruses on it and then touching their mouth or nose.

Is there a vaccine?

There is no widely accepted vaccine, as the genetic makeup of this virus is still being analyzed ,and the vaccine that has been recently approved by FDA did not have enough time (5 years or more) to be tested and to prove it is 100% safe especially for kids and pregnant women!!!!!!

But CDC officials have prepared a "seed stock" of the virus that could be used in the manufacture of a vaccine. Some pharmaceutical companiesare already markettingtheir vaccines!!!!

For swine influenzas that affect pigs, there is a vaccine available that can be given to pigs; there is no vaccine to protect humans from swine flu

I got the flu shot this year. Am I protected ?

Not likely. This is a virus that has never been seen before; therefore, vaccines for human flu would not provide adequate protection from the swine flu material contained in this virus. It may offer some protection though against the human flu genetic elements.

The current outbreak of swine flu that has infected humans is of the H1N1 type - this type is not as dangerous as some others .

Avian Influenza (Bird Flu) can also infect pigs

Avian flu and human seasonal flu viruses can infect pigs, as well as swine influenza. The H3N2 influenza virus subtype, a virulent one, is thought to have come from pigs - it went on to infect humans .

It is possible for pigs to be infected with more than one flu virus subtype simultaneously. When this happens the genes of the viruses have the opportunity to mingle. When different flu subtypes mix they can create a new virus which contains the genes from several sources - a reassortant virus

Although swine influenza tends to just infect pigs, they can, and sometimes do, jump the species barrier and infect humans.

Chapter I

What is the risk for human health?

Outbreaks of human infection from a virus which came from pigs (swine influenza) do happen and are sometimes reported. Symptoms will generally be similar to seasonal human influenzas - this can range from mild or no symptoms at all, to severe and possibly fatal pneumonia .

How dangerous?

In Mexico, more than 100 deaths are suspected from swine flu, but all known cases in the US and elsewhere have been mild. Experts do not know how deadly the flu is, because they do not know how many people have been infected overall.

The new strain seems to be more lethal to those aged 25 to 45 — an ominous sign, as this was a hallmark of the 1918 Spanish flu pandemic that killed tens of millions worldwide.

What is the incubation period?

Only a day or two.

How can you stop the spread?

Standard methods of prevention include covering your mouth when you cough and sneeze. Use tissues and throw them in a bin immediately. Wash your hands often with soap and water. Use alcohol-based hand sanitisers. Avoid sick people. If you become sick, stay home from work or school.

Anyone who has the symptoms should seek medical attention right away. Those who get immediate treatment are most likely going to make a full recovery. Doctors take a nose and throat swab sample to send to the lab for testing. The results will be returned within several days. The treatment is a drug called Tamiflu. The doctor will prescribe Tamiflu if it is needed. Most people will get over the swine flu within just a few days. Once you have had swine flu your body will have an immunity from this particular strain in the future.

What is Swine Flu - H1N1 Virus?

Swine flu, now called H1N1 influenza A, is a type of flu virus. It is a new strain of flu that has just recently been affecting people. It is not caught from pigs or by eating pork. It is a human influenza virus and is being spread by people. It is thought to be a combination of three different flu viruses - swine flu, bird flu and human flu. The new strain is extremely contagious and is quickly spreading across the globe.

H1N1 is different from other strains of influenza. This particular strain of influenza has not been previously exposed to humans before so there are no built up immunities to it. This is what makes it so serious. At the current time there is no preventative drug that you can take in order to avoid getting it. That is why people who are elderly, very young or those who have compromised immune systems must be extremely careful to avoid getting the flu.

Just how dangerous it will be remains to be seen. We are just beginning to see the start of the cases in the United States. It is thought to have originated in Mexico but has since spread globally. The worst cases of it seem to be in Mexico, likely because many people were unaware of the dangers of the flu and did not seek immediate medical treatment.

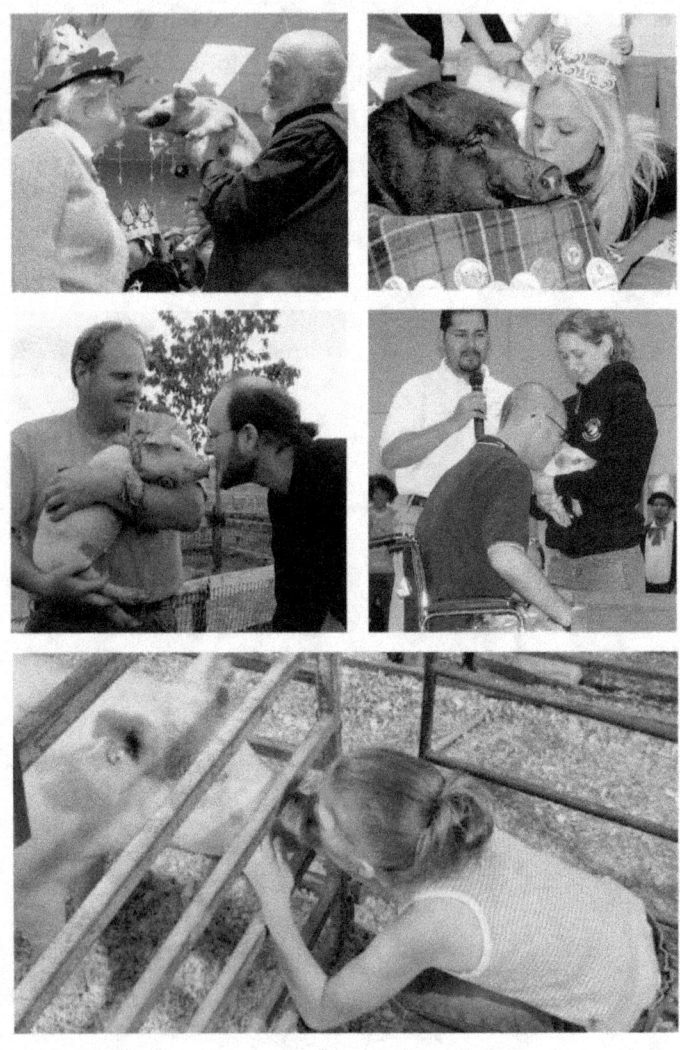

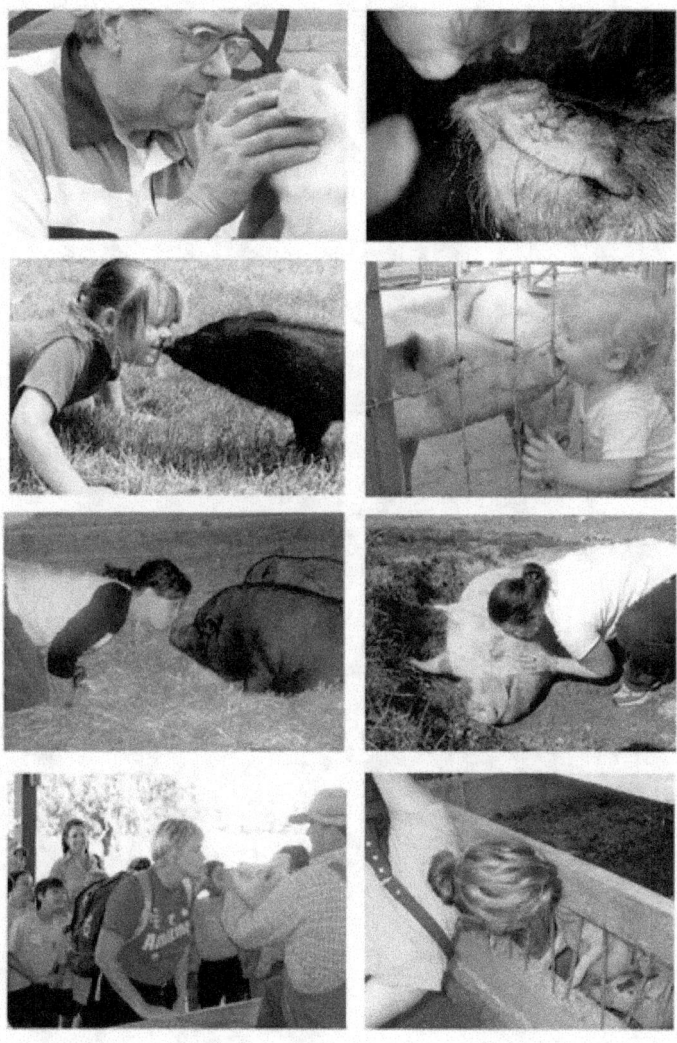

CHAPTER II
Symptoms Of Swine Flu

Swine Flu Symptoms

Swine Flu Basics

Although the name 'swine flu' brings up a lot of extra fear and worry, it is important to note that swine flu is just an influenza A H1N1 virus.

That means that it is just another type of flu virus, just like that which causes our typical seasonal flu symptoms. The big difference is that the current swine influenza A (H1N1) virus has components of pig and bird influenza viruses in it, so that humans don't have any immunity to it. That makes it more likely to become a pandemic virus (have the ability to cause a global outbreak) if it can easily spread from person-to-person.

We do know that swine flu symptoms are just like seasonal flu symptoms:

Swine Flu Symptoms

The symptoms of swine flu are broadly similar to those of ordinary flu, but may be more severe and cause more serious complications:

According to the CDC, like seasonal ordinary flu, symptoms of swine flu infections can include the typical symptoms:

- sudden fever, which is usually high, but unlike seasonal flu, is sometimes absent ;
- sudden cough.
- headache,
- tiredness and fatigue
- chills,

- aching muscles,
- limb or joint pain,
- body aches,
- diarrhea or stomach upset,
- vomiting,
- sore throat,
- runny nose,
- sneezing;
- loss of appetite.

Potentially everyone is at risk from swine flu because few people, if any at all, have enough immunity (resistance) to it.

Signs of a more serious swine flu infection might include pneumonia , respiratory and breathing problems.

If your child has symptoms of swine flu, you should avoid other people and call your pediatrician who might do a rapid flu test to see if he/she has an H1N1 influenza A infection. Further testing can then be done to see if it is a swine flu infection. (Samples are being sent to local and state health departments and the CDC for confirmation of swine flu.)

More Serious Swine Flu Symptoms

More serious symptoms that would indicate that a child with swine flu would need urgent medical attention include:

- Fast breathing or trouble breathing
- Bluish or gray skin color
- Not drinking enough fluids
- Severe or persistent vomiting
- Not waking up or not interacting

- Being so irritable that the child does not want to be held
- Flu-like symptoms improve but then return with high fever and worse cough

Swine Flu Symptoms vs. a Cold or Sinus Infection

It is important to keep in mind most children with a runny nose or cough will not have swine flu and will not have to see their pediatrician for swine flu testing.

This time of year, many other childhood conditions are common, including:

- spring allergies - runny nose, congestion, and cough
- common cold - runny nose, cough, and low grade fever
- sinus infections - lingering runny nose, cough, and fever
- strep throat - sore throat, fever, and a positive strep test

Symptoms of swine flu are like regular flu symptoms and include fever, cough, sore throat, runny nose, body aches, headache, chills, and fatigue. Many people with swine flu have had diarrhea and vomiting. Nearly everyone with flu has at least two of these symptoms. But these symptoms can also be caused by many other conditions. That means that you and your doctor can't know, just based on your symptoms, if you've got swine flu. Health care professionals may offer a rapid flu test, although a negative result doesn't necessarily mean you don't have swine flu.

Only lab tests can definitively show whether you've got swine flu. State health departments can do these tests. But given the large volume of samples coming in to state labs, these tests are being reserved for patients with severe flu symptoms. Currently, doctors are reserving antiviral drugs for people with or at risk of severe flu.

CHAPTER III

Swine Flu And Diabetics

SWINE FLU AND DIABETICS

The best action plan especially for diabetics is to keep your immune system as strong as possible. Diabetics are prone to weak healing from wound and diseases because of a degraded immune system naturally caused by side effects of high blood sugar.

In our contemporary life it is so important to utilize all natural means that provide us with a strong built-in defense with-in our body and be ready for any attack we encounter.

In other books I talked about how GlucoLife can help lower your blood sugar level, but today I want to discuss how some of its ingredients can help you prevent sickness and disease. A strong immune system is what will help save lives if this Swine Flu does spread faster than it can be controlled. Along with lowering your blood sugar here are how ingredients of our product GlucoLife can help BOOST your immune system.

Zinc; this valuable mineral increases the production of white blood cells that fight infection and helps them fight more aggressively.

It also increases natural killer(NK) cells that fight against cancer and helps white cells release more antibodies.

Bitter melon strengthens the immune system, flushes out the toxins in the body. It increases the body`s ability to purify and cleanse impurities hence leading to a more robust immune system

Cinnamon is another wonderful food that improves the immune system.

Alpha Lipoic Acid (ALA): supports a strong immune system and fights damaging free radicals. Alpha lipoic acid supports blood sugar and cholesterol levels, and when used as part of an antioxidant supplement regimen can lead to enhanced wellness.

Fenugreek - It is believed to contain compounds that help relieve inflammation, boost the immune system, and promote liver health. Fenugreek contains powerful antioxidants that help guard healthy cells against damage from free radicals, unstable molecules that attack the body's healthy cells. These antioxidants are natural compounds that seek and destroy free radicals in the body GlucoLife has all of these immunity boosting ingredients visit me at www.pharmatech1.com to find out more

Curcumin, found in abundance in turmeric is an excellent anti-inflammatory agent. Research has shown that its therapeutic activity is equal to other common drugs like Aspirin (NSAIDs) and cortisone. However since it is a natural remedy, curcumin is widely and effectively used to treat diabetes of Type II in India and East Asia and it is well known to have no side effects.

CHAPTER IV

How To Protect Yourself And Your Family From Swine Flu

How To Protect Yourself And Your Family From Swine Flu

What can I do to protect myself?

Stay away from pigs and pig farms.

Wash your hands regularly with soap.

Try to stay healthy.

Get plenty of sleep.

Do plenty of exercise

Try to manage your stress

Drink plenty of liquids

Eat a well balanced diet

Refrain from touching surfaces which may have the virus

Do not get close to people who are sick

Stay away from crowded areas if there is a swine flu outbreak in your area.

All household members should avoid sharing pens, papers, clothes, towels, sheets, blankets, food or eating utensils unless cleaned between uses.

- Disinfect doorknobs, switches, handles, computers, telephones, toys and other surfaces that are commonly touched around the home or workplace.

Wear disposable gloves when in contact with or cleaning up body fluids

If I am infected, how can I stop others from becoming infected?

Limit your contact with other people

Do not go to work or school

When you cough or sneeze cover your mouth with a tissue. If you do not have a tissue, cover your mouth and nose

Put your used tissues in a waste basket

Wash your hands and face regularly

Keep all surfaces you have touched clean

Follow your doctor's instructions

Dr Pickin said there were a number of things that the public could do to assist in restricting the spread of any influenza virus. They include:

1. Wash your hands thoroughly with soap and warm water or use alcohol hand rubs straight after coughing, sneezing or blowing your nose (before touching anything else) and before touching your eyes, nose, mouth, or anything that goes in your mouth.

2. Always carry tissues, and cover a cough or sneeze with a tissue (rather than your hands).

3. Throw used tissues away into suitable containers and perform hand hygiene immediately afterwards.

4. Stand back from other people whenever possible, keeping a distance of at least 1m.

5. Stay at home if you are sick, and minimize contact with other people.

ADDITIONAL FACTS
(May 26,2009)

Dr Pickin says: ``We now know that the H1N1 Influenza 09 virus spreads rapidly, particularly within schools and it is more contagious than seasonal flu.

``The median age for people suffering from the virus is 23 years.

``While most have mild symptoms, the virus does have a hospitalization rate of between 2 and 6%.

``Around half of those who are hospitalised have an underlying condition such as asthma, lung disease or diabetes.

"Around half are people who were previously healthy." .

Can we treat swine flu in humans?

Yes, for the most part. Most of the infections have been treated successfully, though there have been deaths in Mexico and many other countries.

In many cases, patients with this swine flu have recovered on their own. In those who have had to be hospitalized, this virus has been treated with antiviral medications. The virus appears to be week against natural antiviral/antibacterial products.

Here Are Some Tips From The CDC:

- Be sure to continue taking your diabetes pills or insulin. Don't stop taking them even if you can't eat. Your health care provider may even advise you to take more insulin during sickness.

- Test your blood glucose every four hours, and keep track of the results.

- Drink extra (calorie-free) liquids, and try to eat as you normally would. If you can't eat normally, try to ingest soft foods and liquids containing the equivalent amount of carbohydrates that you usually consume.

- Weigh yourself every day. Losing weight without trying to is a sign of high blood glucose.
- Check your temperature every morning and evening. A fever may be a sign of infection.
-

The **CDC** also advises that you call your health care provider or go to an emergency room if any of the following happen to you:

- You feel too sick to eat normally & are unable to keep down food for more than 6 hours.
- You're having severe diarrhea.
- You lose 5 pounds or more.
- Your temperature is over 101 degrees Fahrenheit (38.33 Celsius).
- Your blood glucose is lower than 60 mg/dL or remains over 300 mg/dL.
- You have moderate or large amounts of ketones in your urine.
- You're having trouble breathing.
- You feel sleepy or can't think clearly.

Clean Hands Can Help Save Lives

If things go from bad to worse, it may be difficult to find running water. However, it's still important to wash your hands to avoid illness or infection, especially when testing your blood glucose or treating a wound.

When your hands are visibly dirty, you should wash them with soap and warm water when available. If soap and water are not available, use alcohol-based hand sanitizers.

When should you wash your hands?

- Before preparing or eating food.
- After going to the bathroom.
- After changing diapers or cleaning up a child who has gone to the bathroom.
- Before and after caring for someone who is sick.
- After handling uncooked foods, particularly raw meat, poultry, or fish.
- After blowing your nose, coughing, or sneezing.
- After handling an animal or animal waste.
- After handling garbage.

- Before and after treating a cut or wound.
- After handling items contaminated by flood water or sewage.

CHAPTER V

Swine Flu Conventional Medicines: Is There Any Cure?

Swine Flu Conventional Medicines: Is There Any Cure?

The World Health Organization has rated the UK as one of the best-prepared countries for a swine flu pandemic.

Stocks of antiviral medicines and antibiotics are available to treat anyone who becomes ill during the current pandemic.

Antivirals

One of the ways to lessen the symptoms of pandemic flu is to treat infected people with antiviral medicines, which have been used against the current swine flu. They are not a cure, but will help to:

- reduce the length of time you are ill by around one day,
- relieve some of the symptoms, and
- reduce the potential for serious complications such as pneumonia.

The most famous antiviral medicines used to treat swine flu available in the market are : ***Tamiflu (Oseltamivir) and Ralenza (Zanamivir)***. At the end of this chapter we will talk about the side effects of both drugs.

Antibiotics

Antibiotics will also play an important part in the response to the pandemic. They will be used to treat people in the community if they develop secondary bacterial infections in the lungs, like pneumonia.

In hospitals, antibiotics are used to treat the patients and may reduce the length of hospitalization.

For more information, see the alternative natural antibiotics in the following chapters which are equivalent to 132 chemical antibiotics

Do we need antibiotics in a pandemic?

While antivirals may reduce the number of complications, there are still likely to be significant numbers of complications occurring in the pandemic. Some of the most common include bacterial infections in the respiratory tract and lungs, such as pneumonia. Antibiotics are needed to treat such complications.

Antibiotic-resistant bacteria (pneumonia) could make swine flu far worse

While the talking heads on TV have recently reported that thousands of people in the U.S. are now infected with the new "swine flu", or H1N1, there's another infectious disease problem brewing that has received little attention. The over-use and abuse of antibiotics has produced antibiotic-resistant bacteria. According to the National Institutes of Health, over the past forty years, methicillin-resistant *Staphylococcus aureus* has changed from a usually controllable nuisance into a serious public health problem.

Now a paper just published in the June edition of ***The Lancet Infectious Diseases*** discusses an emerging and potentially deadly threat from community acquired methicillin-resistant *Staphylococcus aureus* (*CA-MRSA*) -- necrotizing, i.e. "flesh eating", pneumonia. And according to previous research published in *Nature News*, this type of pneumonia *is fatal in 75 percent of cases*.

Dr. Hidron and Dr. Blumberg also noted in their paper that, besides causing a high fever, *CA-MRSA* pneumonia can sometimes cause low blood pressure that progresses to septic shock and requires patients to be placed on mechanical respirators in order to breathe. Another important point discussed in the article may turn out to have special relevance due to the emergence of H1N1 influenza, especially by the time flu season rolls around this fall: potentially deadly *CA-MRSA* pneumonia appears to occur most commonly following a flu-type illness.

Does swine flu pose special risks in pregnant women?

During pregnancy, you may have an increased risk of complications from any type of flu, especially in the second and third trimester.

Can women take antiviral drugs during pregnancy?

Though it is not 100% secure and safe some doctors prescribe Tamiflu and Ralenza.

Can children take antivirals?

Even with small doses of Tamiflu or Ralenza it is not 100% secure and safe for infants aged one and older.

Can babies under the age of one take antivirals?

Tamiflu and Ralenza are not licensed for use in babies under the age of one.

Are we more at risk of catching swine flu if I have HIV?

Probably not. Although HIV infects CD4 cells and reduces their number and function, there are other parts of the immune system that are able to fight flu.

Are we more likely to suffer complications if I have HIV and catch swine flu?

If you have a low CD4 count (under 200), you may be more likely to suffer complications like pneumonia from any type of flu, including swine flu.

Can we take antivirals if we have mild to moderate kidney disease?

Yes. But we do recommend to take the 100% safe natural ones.

Are people with asthma or chronic obstructive pulmonary disease (COPD) more at risk from swine flu?

You are no more likely to catch swine flu than anyone else. However, if you do catch a respiratory infection, including swine flu, it may add to the breathing difficulties you may have.

Chapter V

What advice is there for people with asthma or COPD?

We recommend to take a very effective herbal tea mentioned in the following chapters.

Can we take antivirals if we have asthma or COPD?

Yes – We recommend the 100% safe natural ones. However, Ralenza (an inhaler) is usually not given to people with asthma as on rare occasions it can cause breathing complications.

If we have diabetes. Are we at more at risk from swine flu?

We are no more likely to catch swine flu than anyone else. However, if you do catch it, your blood glucose may increase because islet cells partially close and your diabetes treatment may need to be adjusted accordingly.

What should I do if my blood glucose increases because any infection?

Diabetics who take the antibiotic Zithromax (AZITHROMYCIN) were helped by the medication to open the iselet cells and reduce their blood sugar.

Is there any advice for people with liver disease?

If you have liver disease you are no more likely to catch swine flu than anyone else.

Are older people more likely to catch swine flu?

It is not yet known. Almost all of those infected with swine flu in Europe are people under 50 who have recently returned from travel in Mexico. This picture could change.

Are older people more at risk of complications if they do catch it?

Doctors expect that older people are more likely to develop complications from any type of flu, and are generally less able to fight it off but according to published medical reports we see that young people are less resistant against swine flu and its complications since they live on junk food and drinks and therefore they have lower levels of immunity!!!!!!

Why are schools closed for seven days?

The Health Protection Agency has concluded that seven days is the maximum swine flu incubation period - the time between getting the virus and symptoms starting to appear. Schools can reopen earlier than seven days if there is evidence that the suspected case is not swine flu.

Is it safe to use public transport if we were in a pandemic?

Yes. Public transport has not been closed during previous pandemics, and while there is a small additional risk to the public, this is no greater than using other public places. Anyone who has the flu or feels unwell should stay at home and not travel.

Will hospital capacity be adequate?

Most flu sufferers can be cared for appropriately at home if enough care is taken.

Chapter V

Potential Dangers Of Anti-Influenza Drug Tamiflu

Dr. Ben Kim wrote on November 26, 2005:

"I just read a disturbing article in the New York Times about recent reports of deaths and abnormal behaviour in Japanese children who were given the anti-influenza drug Tamiflu.

Here is a summary of the key points I learned from this article:

1. Tamiflu was approved for use in the United States in 1999, and in Japan in late 2000.

2. According to Roche, the manufacturer of Tamiflu, of the 13 million prescriptions written for children worldwide, 11.6 million have been in Japan.

3. According to documents prepared by FDA reviewers, 12 Japanese children, ages 1 to 16, have died after taking Tamiflu. Six of these children, ages 2 to 4, were completely healthy before getting the flu. In the words of the FDA reviewers, "it is concerning that six young patients died suddenly within one to two days after initiation of oseltamivir therapy."

4. Also according to the FDA reviewers, there have been 32 reported instances of "neuropsychiatric events" worldwide, with 31 of them occuring in Japan. These neuropsychiatric events include delirium, abnormal behaviour, and hallucinations.

5. Two Japanese boys, ages 12 and 13, jumped from the second story windows of their homes after receiving two doses of Tamiflu.

6. Two Japanese teenagers who died after receiving Tamiflu are thought to have committed suicide.

7. An 8 year old Japanese boy had a frightening hallucination three hours after receiving his first dose of Tamiflu and rushed into the street outside of his house.

8. There have been multiple reports of severe skin reactions in adults and children all over the world who have taken Tamiflu.

Predictably, Roche has responded to these data by saying that "the reports of these problems were rare given that millions of people had used the drug, and that the problems might have been caused by the flu itself."

Roche has also said that "the death rate among children taking Tamiflu was only one in a million and that the rate of death and other problems was no greater than in children with the flu who did not take the drug."

If this is in fact true, then why take the drug in the first place? If the rates of death for children who take Tamiflu and children who don't take it are the same, why take Tamiflu at all?

"Sorry for the cliche, but no amount of money in this world could persuade me to take Tamiflu or any other flu drug or vaccine. And you better believe that I'd do everything I possibly could to make sure that my own child is never exposed to such drugs. It amazes and saddens me to know that so many children and adults all over the world take drugs like Tamiflu thinking that they are perfectly safe and that they are doing something good for their health."(**by Charles Choi,UPI Science News**)

Chapter V

From Reuters Health:

U.S. FDA, Roche warn on Tamiflu dangers:

Last Updated: 2008-03-04 14:14:08 -0400 (Reuters Health)

WASHINGTON (Reuters) - U.S. regulators and Roche Holding AG have warned doctors of psychiatric events, some of which resulted in death, in patients taking the flu drug Tamiflu (oseltamivir), regulators said on Tuesday.

Drugmaker Roche wrote a letter, dated February 2008, to health professionals advising them of a recent update to the Tamiflu label, according to a notice posted on the Food and Drug Administration's Web site.

The revised label includes a new description of reports of delirium and other abnormal behavior, with some cases resulting in fatal outcomes, the letter said. The previous language did not mention any deaths.

The new label says the cases "appear to be uncommon" and "the contribution of Tamiflu to these events has not been established."

The company said the revisions reflect recommendations made in November 2007 by an FDA advisory panel that reviewed the cases, which have been seen mostly in Japan.

"The changes to the label reflect observations from a growing body of data, which shows no evidence of a causal relationship between Tamiflu and the reported adverse events," Roche said in a statement.

The new label also notes influenza itself can be associated with various psychiatric problems.

Copyright Reuters 2009.

Very Important Comment:

It is well known that Tamiflu was designed and approved by FDA to be used for Avian(bird) flu and to be approved for swine flu it does need to enter all steps , phases and double blind studies before it is allowed to be an official prescription for swine flu!!!!!!

CHAPTER VI

Warning: Swine Flu Vaccine Coming Soon

Warning: Swine Flu Vaccine Coming Soon

Specialty drug maker Baxter International Inc. says it's in "full scale" production of a swine flu vaccine. The vaccine will be commercially available in July .

The company made its announcement one day after the World Health Organization declared swine flu a global pandemic .

The U.S. Centers for Disease Control and Prevention (CDC) reports 45 swine flu deaths nationwide.

The National Vaccine Information Center will hold its 4th conference in Washington DC October 2-4 of this year. I will be speaking there as will some of the leading experts in vaccines in the world. Clearly the best vaccine conference in the world and it is only held every few years. If this is of any interest to you I would strongly encourage you to attend.

Sources : Washington Post June 13, 2009

National Vaccine Information Center (NVIC) June 18, 2009

Dr. Mercola's Comments :

"As I predicted in my first swine flu alert, a fast-tracked swine flu vaccine was promptly ordered, and will be available as early as July. Pharmaceutical giant Baxter claims it has patented technology that cuts the usual vaccine development time in half, to about 13 weeks instead of 26 .

Although many governments and health organizations are probably celebrating this feat, you have no reason to join in the festivities. In fact, you have good reason to fear being exposed to this new swine flu vaccine more than the swine flu itself.

You are virtually guaranteed that no safety evaluations will be performed prior to the reckless unleashing of this untested vaccine .

And, making matters worse, your children may be the first guinea pigs in this public vaccine experiment against a previously unseen hybrid of human, bird and pig viruses.

School Children May Face Mandatory Swine Flu Vaccinations

I was hoping mandatory vaccinations would not happen, but it now appears as though that's exactly what we might be facing in the near future .

In the video above, Barbara Loe Fisher of the National Vaccine Information Center (NVIC) warns that there is a campaign underway to turn schools into virtual vaccination clinics, and children will be the first to be injected with experimental swine flu vaccines .

Part of the reasoning for this is that it appears people over the age of 50 have more cross-reacting antibodies against the current swine flu virus, whereas children who have never been exposed to any of the strains before are more vulnerable."

The Post Gazette recently reported experts saying, "if the new H1N1 flu comes back in force this fall, it might be better to vaccinate children first," because "in the early stages of the epidemic this spring, the new flu strain has caused "explosive outbreaks" among schoolchildren who have no immunity to it".

Again, it's troubling to see health officials using the term "explosive outbreaks" for a flu that in the vast majority of cases has been reported to be very mild .

Such inflammatory language is simply uncalled for .

Making matters worse, they want to target children who have underlying health problems, i.e. the most vulnerable of the group, which means any potential problems with this untested vaccine will have the capacity to do maximum damage.

Why are We Putting Up With the Same Mistakes Again?

The current evolution of public health decisions has disturbing similarities to previous swine flu vaccine catastrophes'. The last swine flu threat emerged in 1976, right before I entered medical school and I remember it very clearly. It resulted in the massive swine flu vaccine campaign .

However, within a few months, claims totalling $1.3 billion had been filed by victims who had suffered paralysis from the experimental vaccine. Several hundred people developed crippling Guillain-Barré Syndrome after their injections. Even healthy 20-year-olds ended up as paraplegics. The vaccine was also blamed for 25 deaths .

Meanwhile, the deadly swine flu pandemic itself NEVER materialized…

When a vaccine is developed in a mere 13 weeks, you can be virtually assured that it has NOT had the time to be tested in clinical trials to determine safety and effectiveness .

The way I see it, we now stand poised to experience a repeat of the last dangerous swine flu vaccine, which destroyed the lives of hundreds of healthy young boys and girls .

The real kicker, of course, is the fact that if the new vaccine turns out to be a killer, the pharmaceutical companies responsible have immunity from any lawsuits -- something I've also warned about before on numerous occasions .

Absolutely no one stands to be liable if this vaccine turns out to be a health disaster.

Governments Take Unnecessary "Code Red" Attitude to Flu Threat

The U.S. Congress handed over unprecedented power to the Centers for Disease Control (CDC) after 9-11, and they're chomping at the bit to exercise it now that the World Health Organization (WHO) has upgraded the swine flu threat to Phase 6, Pandemic status .

But really, the word 'pandemic' only means that a new virus is spreading across the world. It says nothing about its level of physical danger .

So far, the swine flu has claimed a mere 332 lives WORLDWIDE (as of July 1), 116 of the deaths occurred in Mexico.

To keep this in perspective, the regular flu (not the swine flu) has allegedly killed 13,000 in the U.S. since January, although there is strong support that these types of figures are grossly exaggerated to increase vaccine sales. However, the fact remains that the regular flu at this point in time is FAR more dangerous than the swine flu, and were you worried about the regular flu before the media started hyping up this exotic new "killer flu ؟"

Despite the indications that the swine flu is more a pandemic nuisance than a pandemic killer, the U.S. Congress responded to the CDC's public health emergency declaration by handing over one billion dollars to a group of drug companies, including Baxter, to fast track experimental swine flu vaccines that may include whole live, dead, or genetically engineered human and animal flu viruses .

Additionally, nearly all vaccines contain a variety of adjuvants – potentially dangerous chemicals used as preservatives and/or to boost the vaccine's potency by affecting your immune system, such as thimerosal.

But the 'code red' attitude to this phantom threat doesn't end there .

Barbara Loe Fisher warns in her article ‹

"In some states, like Massachusetts, public health doctors have persuaded legislators to quickly pass pandemic influenza legislation that will allow state officials to enter the homes and businesses without the approval of occupants; to investigate and quarantine individuals without their consent;

to require licensed health care providers to give citizens vaccines and to ban the free assembly of citizens in the state".

Banning free assembly?

Clearly our law-makers are wise enough to foresee public outcry in the face of forced mass-vaccinations, even if they can't see the insanity behind their legislations to begin with.

What Can You Do ?

I urge you to review the vast supply of information available on the NVIC site, and join Barbara Loe Fisher in her urging to take action against the potential threat of mandatory swine flu vaccinations.

It's imperative that you educate yourself about vaccinations, influenza, vaccine risks, and the public health laws in your state, so you know what you're up against come the beginning of the new school year.

You need to find out what your rights and options are under new public health laws that may require you and your children to get vaccinated or be quarantined.

Many do not realize that such laws even exist. But the Model State Emergency Health Powers Act (MSEHPA), which was passed by many states in 2002, includes provisions that would allow state health officials to use the state militia to:

Take control of all roads leading into and out of cities and states;

Seize homes, cars, telephones, computers, food, fuel, clothing, firearms and alcoholic beverages for their own use (and not be held liable if these actions result in the destruction of personal property(. Arrest, imprison and forcibly examine, vaccinate and medicate citizens without consent) and not be held liable if these actions result in your death or injury. **Take Action Now**

I recommend you visit www.NVIC.org and learn as much as you can .

Says Fisher:

"As Department of Homeland Security officials are declaring that any disease outbreak is a matter of homeland security; as Department of Defense officials are defining public demonstrations as "low level terrorism; as CDC officials make plans to re-route airplanes to designated airports with quarantine centers to screen all passengers for signs of swine flu.;as fast tracked experimental pandemic flu vaccines are being created to be given to American children first, it is time for all of us – whether we are public health officials addressing what we believe is a true public health emergency or whether we are ordinary citizens simply trying to protect our health and the health of our children - to act in rational and responsible ways".

I agree .

This is not the time to fall for hype. These public scare-tactics are designed to make money, not protect your health.

You can also register to attend the Fourth International Public Conference on Vaccination Oct. 2-4, 2009 in Washington, D.C. and help organize in your state to protect your right to informed consent to vaccination .

Also, call and write your state legislators. Let them know where you stand on these issues .

How to Protect Yourself without Dangerous Drugs and Vaccinations?

Last but not least, let me reiterate the many ways you can protect your health from ANY kind of flu, without a potentially dangerous vaccine.

I have not caught a flu in over two decades, and you can avoid it too by following these simple guidelines, which will keep your immune system in optimal working order so that you're far less likely to acquire the infection to begin with .

1-Optimize your vitamin D levels. As I've previously reported, optimizing your vitamin D levels is one of the absolute best strategies for avoiding infections of ALL kinds, and vitamin D deficiency is likely the TRUE culprit behind the seasonality of the flu -- not the flu virus itself .

I would STRONGLY urge you to have your vitamin D level monitored to confirm your levels are therapeutic at 50-70 ng.ml and done by a reliable vitamin D lab like Lab Corp .

If you are coming down with flu like symptoms and have not been on vitamin D you can take doses of 50,000 units a day for three days to treat the acute infection. Some researchers like Dr. Cannell, believe the dose could even be as high as 1,000 units per pound of body weight for three days.

However, most of Dr. Cannell's work was with seasonal and not pandemic flu. If your body has never been exposed to the antigens there is chance that the vitamin D might not work. Your best bet is to maintain healthy levels of vitamin D around 60 ng/ml.

2-Avoid Sugar and Processed Foods. Sugar decreases the function of your immune system almost immediately, and as you likely know, a strong immune system is key to fighting off viruses and other illness. Remember that sugar is present in foods you may not suspect, like ketchup and fruit juice.

3-Get Enough Rest. Just like it becomes harder for you to get your daily tasks done if you're tired, if your body is overly fatigued it will be harder for it to fight the flu. Be sure to check out my article Guide to a Good Night's Sleep for some great tips to help you get quality rest .

4-Have Effective Tools to Address Stress. We all face some stress every day, but if stress becomes overwhelming then your body will be less able to fight off the flu and other illness .

If you feel that stress is taking a toll on your health, consider using a tool such as meridian tapping techniques, which is remarkably effective in relieving stress associated with all kinds of events, from work to family to trauma. You can check out my free, 25-page manual for some guidelines on how to perform this simple technique .

5-Exercise. When you exercise, you increase your circulation and your blood flow throughout your body. The components of your immune system are also better circulated, which means your immune system has a better chance of finding an illness before it spreads. You can review my exercise guidelines for some great tips on how to get started .

6-Take a good source of animal-based omega-3 fats like krill oil. Increase your intake of healthy and essential fats like the omega-3 found in krill oil, which is crucial for maintaining health. It is also vitally important to avoid damaged omega-6 oils like trans fats as it will seriously damage your immune response.

7-Wash Your Hands. Washing your hands will decrease your likelihood of spreading a virus to your nose, mouth or to other people. Be sure you don't use antibacterial soap for this -- antibacterial soaps are completely unnecessary, and they cause far more harm than good. Instead, identify a simple chemical-free soap that you can switch your family to.

8-Use All-Natural 'Antibiotics'.Garlic works like a broad-spectrum antibiotic against bacteria,virus, and protozoa in your body. And unlike synthetic antibiotics, no resistance can be built up so it is an absolutely safe product to use. However, if you are allergic or don't enjoy garlic it would be best to avoid as it will likely cause more harm than good.

Other all-natural antibiotics include olive leaf extract and oil of oregano .

I will avoid Hospitals and Vaccines in this particular case, and will stay away from hospitals unless I have an emergency, as hospitals may be prime breeding grounds for infections of all kinds, and could be one of the likeliest places you could be exposed to this new bug .

Related Links : Critical Alert: The Swine Flu Pandemic – Fact or Fiction?

CHAPTER VII
Herbs To Raise WBC,CD4 And Immunity

Herbs To Raise WBC,CD4 And Immunity

From Wikipedia, the free encyclopedia

White blood cells (WBCs), or **leukocytes** are cells of the immune system defending the body against both infectious disease and foreign materials.

The number of leukocytes in the blood is often an indicator of disease. There are normally between 4×10^9 and 1.1×10^{10} white blood cells in a liter of blood.

WBC regulates the body's **immune system**, identifying, fighting and engulfing germs. It is also essential to life, since we are literally surrounded by **bacteria, fungi, viruses and protozoa** (all "germs") which would take over our bodies and kill us if we did not have an immunee system to fight them off and this is the major role of WBC.

CD4 tests measure the number of T cells containing the CD4 receptor. Results are usually expressed in the number of cells per microliter (or mm^3) of blood. CD4 are used to assess the immune system of patients. Patients often undergo treatments when the **CD4** count reaches a low point, around 200 cells per microliter. Medical professionals also refer **to** **CD4** tests to determine the efficacy of the treatment. For example; in HIV/AIDS patients if viral load becomes zero and **CD4** more than 500 then we say he/she is OK.

To enhance immunity against any bacterial or viral attack we need to take natural herbs to increase both WBC and CD4.

WBC increasing herbs

Myrrh: research papers show that Myrrh increases WBC

Berberine (Goldenseal) exhibits potent anticancer activity directly by killing tumor cells and indirectly via stimulating white blood cells (**WBC**).

Uses and Benefits: Goldenseal is marketed as a tonic and natural antibiotic, and it is often combined with echinacea to help "strengthen the immune system." As a popular American folk medicine, goldenseal has been used as an antiseptic, astringent, or hemostatic to treat a wide variety of skin, eye, and mucous membrane inflammatory and infectious conditions. Thus, it has been employed as a mouthwash, for canker sores, and as a topical agent for dermatologic disorders. Some herbalists also view goldenseal as a mucous membrane "alternative"-increasing and decreasing mucus secretion depending on the body's needs.

Echinacea increases the white blood cell count when it is deficient

Ginseng: Ginseng has been shown to have different effects on immune effector cells and cytokine levels in laboratory, animal and human studies .

Astragalus: Astragalus increases CD4/CD8 ratio and enhances immunity.

Cayenne and vinegar credited with increasing **CD4**, CD8 and **WBC** counts

Cd4 Increasing Herbs:

- **Black walnut Extract**
- **Wormwood from the Artemesia shrub**
- **Cloves from the clove tree**
- **Arginine Amino Acid**
- **Licorice Extract.**
- **Melatonin**
- **Alpha Lipoic acid 25mg**
- **Acetyl-L-Carnitine 250mg 1/4 to 1/2 capsule**
- **Green Tea**
- **Grape seed**
- **Olive Leaf Extract**
- **Grapefruit Seed**
- **Pumpkin Seed**

- **Reishi Mushroom Extracts**
- **Agaricus blazei Brasilian Mushroom**
- **Shiitake Mushroom**

LITHIUM CARBONATE : It increases WBC too.

Burdock Root: an excellent blood cleanser and immunity stimulant for cold and flu.

Zizyphus jujube

Lycii Fruit: Research shows that **Lycii Berry** Improves Memory, Enhances Immune Function, and Increases Stamina. Related topics include Memory Loss, Alzheimer's, and Fatigue

CURCUMIN is an excellent immunity enhancer in a new study.

Apple Cider Vinegar

Colostrum increases CD4 counts (reported).

Whole Lemon/Olive Oil drink daily

Andrographis herb found that while it tended to decrease viral load and increase **CD4** lymphocyte levels in people with HIV infection!!!

Phytosterols/sterolins have been demonstrated elsewhere to selectively increase CD4 and lymphocyte counts. The sterol content in many plants are thought to be one of the major chemical compounds contributing to the health benefits of a variety of medicinal herbs such as Saw Palmetto, Pygeum, Pumpkin seeds, Devil's Claw, Milk Thistle, Ginkgo Biloba, Panax and Siberian Ginseng .

Neem tree has both pesticidal and medicinal properties .

Aloe Vera: an excellent immune stimulant and used extensively for cancer and other immunity disorder diseases.

Selenium : used for AIDS ,cancer and hepatitis B and C as an immunity enhancer.

Zinc:

Zinc is necessary for the functioning of over 300 different enzymes and plays a vital role in an enormous number of biological processes.

Zinc is a cofactor for the antioxidant enzyme superoxide dismutase (SOD) and is in a number of enzymatic reactions involved in carbohydrate and protein metabolism.

Its immunologic activities include regulation of T lymphocytes, CD4، natural killer cells, and interleukin II. In addition, **zinc has been claimed to possess antiviral activity**. It has been shown to play a role in wound healing, especially following burns or surgical incisions. Zinc is necessary for the maturation of sperm and normal fetal development. It is involved in sensory perception (taste, smell‹and vision) and controls the release of stored vitamin A from the liver. Within the endocrine system, zinc has been shown to regulate insulin activity and promote the conversion of thyroid hormones, thyroxin, into tri-iodothyronine.

Based on available scientific evidence, zinc may be efficacious in the treatment of (childhood) malnutrition, acne vulgaris, peptic ulcers‹ leg ulcers, infertility, Wilson's disease, herpes, and taste or smell disorders. Zinc has also gained popularity for its use in prevention of the common cold.

Zinc appears to be an essential trace element for the immune system.

CHAPTER VIII

The Healing Powers of sex
For Immune System

The Healing Powers of sex
For Enhancing Immune System

Sex is not only the most significant aspect of any successful romantic relationship but also has tremendous healing potential. In a recent study, it was revealed that individuals who indulged in regular sexual activities stayed healthier and lived longer than those who refrained from having sex!!!!!

This proves that sex not only gives you pleasure but is also a great remedy for battling an array of ailments ranging from heart disease, obesity and depression to skin disorders, stress and even cancer

Bust stress with sex:

Various modern day studies have revealed that sex is an amazing stress buster that helps lower the elevated stress levels of the body and enables you to live a happier and healthier life. Individuals having sex frequently tend to have a better response towards daily life stressors than those who abstain from it or lead a celibate lifestyle.

A big health benefit of sex is lower blood pressure and overall stress reduction, according to researchers from

Scotland who reported their findings in the journal *Biological Psychology*. They studied 24 women and 22 men who kept records of their sexual activity. Then the researchers subjected them to stressful situations -- such as speaking in public and doing verbal arithmetic -- and noted their blood pressure response to stress.

Sex for enhancing your body's Immunity:

Good sexual health may mean better physical health. Having sex once or twice a week has been linked with higher levels of an antibody called immunoglobulin A or IgA, which can protect you from getting colds and other infections. Scientists at Wilkes University in Wilkes-Barre, Pa., took samples of saliva, which contain IgA, from 112 college students who reported the frequency of sex they had

Those in the "frequent" group -- once or twice a week -- had higher levels of IgA than those in the other three groups -- who reported being abstinent, having sex less than once a week, or having it very often, three or more times weekly.

Sex can certainly boost your immune system and may even prevent you from catching cold and all types of flu including Swine Flu.

This is because having regular sex increases the levels of immunoglobulin A, an antibody. Individuals who regularly indulge in sex have higher levels of this antibody than those who rarely have sex!!!!

IT'S OFFICIAL! Sex is good for your health.

American health experts reckon sex is one of the best ways to fight off winter cold and flu bugs.

And their study suggests that people who aren't getting enough could be left feeling down in more ways than one.

Professor Carl Charnetski reckons that having sex twice a week is the perfect medicine for the common cold.

"We found that individuals engaging in sex once or twice a week have substantially higher levels of antibodies than those reporting no sexual activity," he said.

His study found that having sex raised levels of the immunity.

Burn calories with sex:

Sex is considered to be one of the best forms of exercise. As per research, about 30 minutes of great sex can lead to burning 85 calories. A single session of sex is equivalent to around 20 laps of swimming and it also helps tone up your body muscles and enhances the flow of oxygen and blood to all body parts.

Thirty minutes of sex burns 85 calories or more. It may not sound like much, but it adds up: 42 half-hour sessions will burn 3,570 calories, more than enough to lose a pound. Doubling up, you could drop that pound in 21 hour-long sessions.

"Sex is a great mode of exercise," says Patti Britton, PhD, a Los Angeles sexologist and president of the American Association of Sexuality Educators and Therapists. It takes work, from both a physical and psychological perspective, to do it well, she says.

Sex combats depression:

Sex is one of the best known tranquilizers for treating mild cases of depression. This is because when you have sex, the happy hormones or endorphins are released that are known to promote feelings of happiness and well being. Studies tell us that sex is 10 times more potent than Valium when it comes to treating depression and has no side effects

Sex helps you sleep better and solves the insomnia problem:

A compound known as oxytocinis released while having sex. This is known to promote sound sleep. Sex is considered to be highly relaxing and eases the tension from every muscle of your body. It enables you to fall asleep with ease and is much safer than all those harmful sleeping pills available in the market.

The oxytocin released during orgasm also promotes sleep, according to research.

And getting enough sleep has been linked with a host of other good things, such as maintaining a healthy weight and blood pressure. Something to think about, especially if you've been wondering why your guy can be active one minute and snoring the next.

Sex Improves Cardiovascular Health

While some older folks may worry that the efforts expended during sex could cause a stroke, that's not so, according to researchers from England. In a study published in the *Journal of Epidemiology and Community Health*, scientists found frequency of sex was not associated with stroke in the 914 men they followed for 20 years.

And the heart health benefits of sex don't end there. The researchers also found that having sex twice or more a week reduced the risk of fatal heart attack by half for the men, compared with those who had sex less than once a month.

Sex Boosts Self-Esteem

Boosting self-esteem was one of 237 reasons people have sex, collected by University of Texas researchers and published in the *Archives of Sexual Behavior.*

That finding makes sense to Gina Ogden, PhD, a sex therapist and marriage and family therapist in Cambridge, Mass., although she finds that those who already have self-esteem say they sometimes have sex to feel even better. "One of the reasons people say they have sex is to feel good about themselves," she tells WebMD. "Great sex begins with self-esteem, and it raises it. If the sex is loving, connected, and what you want, it raises it."

Sex Improves Intimacy

Having sex and orgasms increases levels of the hormone oxytocin, the so-called love hormone, which helps us bond and build trust. Researchers from the University of Pittsburgh and the University of North Carolina evaluated 59 premenopausal women before and after warm contact with their husbands and partners ending with hugs. They found that the more contact, the higher the oxytocin levels.

"Oxytocin allows us to feel the urge to nurture and to bond," Britton says.

Higher oxytocin has also been linked with a feeling of generosity. So if you're feeling suddenly more generous toward your partner than usual, credit the love hormone.

Sex Reduces Pain

As the hormone oxytocin surges, endorphins increase, and pain declines. So if your headache, arthritis pain, or PMS symptoms seem to improve after sex, you can thank those higher oxytocin levels.

In a study published in the *Bulletin of Experimental Biology and Medicine,* 48 volunteers who inhaled oxytocin vapor and then had their fingers pricked lowered their pain threshold by more than half.

Sex Reduces Prostate Cancer Risk

Frequent ejaculations, especially in 20-something men, may reduce the risk of prostate cancer later in life, Australian researchers reported in the *British Journal of Urology International.* When they followed men diagnosed with prostate cancer and those without, they found no association of prostate cancer with the number of sexual partners as the men reached their 30s, 40s, and 50s.

But they found men who had five or more ejaculations weekly while in their 20s reduced their risk of getting prostate cancer later by a third.

Another study, reported in the *Journal of the American Medical Association*, found that frequent ejaculations, 21 or more a month, were linked to lower prostate cancer risk in older men, as well, compared with less frequent ejaculations of four to seven monthly.

Sex Strengthens Pelvic Floor Muscles

For women, doing a few pelvic floor muscle exercises known as Kegels during sex offers a couple of benefits. You will enjoy more pleasure, and you'll also strengthen the area and help to minimize the risk of incontinence later in life.

To do a basic Kegel exercise, tighten the muscles of your pelvic floor, as if you're trying to stop the flow of urine. Count to three, then release.

Sex Improves Blood Circulation and Enhances Memory:

Mental stimulation improves brain function and actually protects against cognitive decline, as does physical exercise. The human brain is able to continually adapt and rewire itself. Even in old age, it can grow new neurons. Severe mental decline is usually caused by disease, whereas most age-related losses in memory or motor skills simply result from inactivity and a lack of mental exercise and stimulation.

In other words, use it or lose it. Walking is especially good for your brain, because it increases blood circulation and the oxygen and glucose that reach your brain running also leads to increased brain cell numbers in normal adult and elderly "senior citizen". Even sex helps to increase blood flow to the brain.

Our clinic at Yrmouk University tested the effect of sex(intercourse and kissing) on huge number of cases for different conditions and all results showed that sex has a great positive effect based on reducing stress, hypertension and enhancing immunity.

I myself tested its effect on my high blood pressure together with my product **PRESS OIL** *which is composed of a number of essential oils and works as a natural external* **vasodilator** *and Iam now hypertension free since March 2008!!!*

For more information about this topic please visit:
(ayurvediccure.com and.webmd.com)

CHAPTER IX
pH, Acidity, Alkalinity and Swine Flu

pH, Acidity, Alkalinity and Swine Flu

Most people have a good understanding that eating healthy foods will help in keeping them fit and resistant to flu viruses. What they may not know is that their body has an **acid/alkaline balance** that when shifted can leave them prone to sicknesses. With the rise of the pandemic outbreak of the swine flu virus, you will want to know how to prepare yourself and your family to resist it and the potential dangers it carries.

Steps to be more healthy with Acid/Alkaline Balance

Step 1: Understand what pH, or potential of hydrogen means and why it is significant. Everything around us carries a value on this scale ranging from 1 to 14 with 7 as being neutral and 1 being very acid. Our body fluids prefer to be slightly alkaline in the range of about 7.4. At this point, the oxygen level is higher than the hydrogen level and aerobic metabolism is carried out.

Test yourself by getting some simple pH testing strips available at local drug stores or online. If you test both your urine and saliva Ph you can average them out to get a decent reading. Compare them with the chart on the container to see where your pH reads.

Adjust your diet so that the foods you eat are contributing to either increase your alkalinity or acidity, depending on the outcome of

Step 2: Green leafy foods are generally highly alkaline but lemons and watermelon are alkaline. We can quickly correct the acid balance, along with hundreds of other foods. Most people will tend to be too acidic rather than too alkaline but looking at the chart of acid/alkaline foods can guide you to the right choices. Generally, bright colored foods are not only delicious but very alkaline acting in your body.

It is recommended to go Alkaline in food and drinks if you have any type of flu:

Alkaline Food/Drink Examples:

- **Vitamin C**:. boosts the immunity and taking 1000mgs of vitamin C on regular basis can prevent colds and flus. Take vitamin C with Curcumin will prevent both cold and flu.

- **Zinc** is used to enhance the immune system against colds and flu viruses as we discussed in a previous chapter.

- **Vitamin A** protects the integrity of mucus membranes and helps prevent infections. Other than taking the RDA of vitamin A in a multivitamin it is not advisable to take extra vitamin A. Just try eating foods rich in vitamin A like carrots, spinach, red peppers, and sweet potatoes.

- **Calcium.** Getting the right amount of calcium in the diet can help the immune system by boosting the alkalinity of the body. Viruses, bad bacteria, and other body invaders thrive in more acidic environments. Making the body more alkaline can aid in weakening the cold virus. Take no more than the RDA of calcium. For most people it is around 1500mgs. One great way to get calcium during a cold is to drink calcium fortified orange juice.

Foods that boost the immune system.

Eating some foods may help resist colds, and flu such as:

Garlic is an immune enhancing agent with anti-inflammatory properties .

Baking Powder is one of the best alkaline foods and a glass of water with a spoon of powder can kill all types of viruses including swine flu virus (see chapter 10)

Apple: one of the best immunity enhancing alkaline foods which helps against cold and flu. Moreover it is recommended to take one apple in the morning instead of coffee or tea.

An apple a day keeps cold and flu away!!!!!

CHAPTER X

Prof.Mansour Swine Flu Protocol

PROF.MANSOUR SWINE FLU PROTOCOL

SPECIFICS:

Swine flu is a highly contagious viral infection of the respiratory tract and is spread by coughing and sneezing. Symptoms include headache, fever, aching of limbs and back, and weakness.

(Beneficial Remedies, Treatments, and Nutrients)

HERBALCOMBINATIONS:

(*FLU TECH HERBAL TEA OR CAPSULES FORMULA*)

PHYSIOLOGICAL ACTION:

Proven herbal formulas to help relieve symptoms of colds, flu, hoarseness, colic, high fevers and germinal viral infections. Herbal Influence was created with herbs which help with fever , nausea and vomiting symptoms.

SINGLE HERBS:

Andrographis Paniculata, Propolis,Cayenne, Echinacea , Red Clover, Raspberry Leaf, Chaparral, Rose Hips, Garlic,

Honey, Turkish Rhubarb, and Golden Seal, Olive Leaf, Mastic Leaf, Elderberry

HERBAL TEA :

TERMINALIA CHEBULA TEA ,AINSE TEA, VIOLET TEA ,WILD CHERRY BARK, RASBERRY TEA

VITAMINS: D3, C, B complex

AMINO ACIDS: L-Lysine has a direct effect on the virus

MINERALS: Zinc, Multi-Mineral Complex.

DRINKS: Camel Milk ,Fulvic Herbal Drink, Lemon-Mint Juice,Licorice Infused-Juice

HELPFUL FOODS: :Honey, Amla Fruit, Aloe Vera ,**Mamey** Apples, Apricots, Cherries, Citrus Fruits, Broccoli, Carrots, Green Leafy, Terminalia Chebula Fruit,Mastic Gum

Details of the Major Herbs of the Protocol Secrets:

Tamiflu chemical drug is based on **Shikimic Acid** which is found in Anise and many other plants ,fruits and herbs;

PLANTS CONTAINING SHIKIMIC ACID:

Here is the list of the phytochemical plants containing

Shikimic Acid according to concentration:

1-Mamey Fruit Leaf:

It is a tropical fruit native to South and Central America and it is used in different drinks, ice cream in Peurto Rico and Florida.

Mamey Apricot Leaf contains **700,000 ppm of Shikimic Acid** which is the active ingredient of Tamiflu.

Mamey Apricot Leaf has a strong anti-bacterial , anti-viral and anti-oxidant properties and used for different viral diseases .It is good to know that **Mamey is an evergreen tree!!!!**

In Santo Domingo, the seed kernel oil is used as a skin ointment and as a hair dressing believed to stop falling hair. The oil is employed as a sedative in eye and ear ailments. A seed infusion is used as an eyewash in Cuba. In Mexico, the pulverized seed coat is reported to be a remedy for coronary trouble and is said to be helpful against kidney stones and rheumatism. The Aztecs employed it against epilepsy. The seed kernel is regarded as a digestive; the oil is said to be diuretic. In Costa Rica a "tea" of the bark and leaves is administered in arteriosclerosis and hypertension. Therefore Tamey Tea(TT) offers you a number of health benefits besides swine flu.

2- Terminalia Chebula Fruit:

Its paste with water is found to be anti-inflammatory, analgesic and having healing effects for wounds. Its decoction as a lotion is surgical dressing for healing the wound earlier.

These are used for astringent purpose in hemorrhoids as well. Its decoction is used as gargle in oral ulcers, and sore throat.

Terminalia Chebula & Abdominal Disorders:

It is good to increase the appetite, as digestive aid, liver stimulant, as stomachic, and excellent agent for ulcerative colitis.

It stimulates the liver and protects it further by expelling the waste excretory products from the intestines.

The powder of Terminalia Chebula has been used in chronic diarrahea with excellent results.

For persons with excessive gas in intestine, flatulence, it is an excellent herb that can be taken daily. It relieves these conditions smoothly.

One compound Chebulagic acid from terminalia chebula has shown excellent antispasmodic action .

Being a mild laxative, it is a mild herbal colon cleanser. With its other properties, it provides some help in conditions with liver and spleen enlargement and in ascites. Moreover it can be taken for a long time without any side effects.

Chapter X

Terminalia Chebula & Central Nervous System:

It is a good nervine. It is used in nervous weakness, nervous irritability. It promotes the receiving power of the five senses.

Terminalia Chebula For Heart & Blood Vessels:

It is adjuvant in hemorrhages due to its astringent nature. It helps in edema and various inflammations.

Terminalia Chebula For Lungs & Airways Pulmonary Disorders:

It is good for Chronic Cough, sore throat and bronchial asthma.

Terminalia Chebula For Reproductive Or Sexual Health:

Being anti-inflammatory, and astringent, it is useful in urethral discharges like vaginal discharges .

Terminalia Chebula For Kidney & Urinary Bladder:

It is helpful in Renal calculi, and retention of urine.

Terminalia Chebula For Skin Disorders:

It is useful in skin disorders with discharges like allergies

,and urticaria.

General Uses Of Terminalia Chebula:

It is given as adjuvant herb in chronic fever.

Anti-Bacterial and Antioxidant Properties

Some preliminary evidence of its capability to be useful in HSV Herpes simplex virus. Some anti-tumor activity and effect in inhibiting the HIV virus.Wide Antibacterial and antifungal activity, especially against E. coli.

Based on the many collective health benefits of Terminalia Chebula Fruit and the high content of **Shikimic Acid(22,000 ppm) it is highly recommended for swine flu and its symptoms especially in India and East Asia where it abundant.**

3- Pistacia Lentiscus L.(Mastic Tree)Leaf:

Mastic Is More Than An Antibacterial!!!!

Mastic gum and leaf have strong anti-bacterial and antiviral properties and it is considered one of the strongest natural weapons against H.Pylori the most dangerous bacteria which causes stomach ulcer and cancer, colon cancer and many auto-immune diseases such as arthritis, diabetes and lupus!!!!!

Mastic Leaf contains 18,000 ppm of **Shikimic Acid** .

Mastic tree is evergreen tree found in Greece, France, Turkey, Palestine and Syria. It is also available in some Asian , African and American countries.

4- Opuntia ficus-indica (L.) -- Indian Fig, Nopal, Prickly Pear Fruit:

Prickly pears are members of the cactus family, which includes about 97 genera and 1,600 species. The species are found in Europe, Mediterranean countries, Africa, South Western countries, United States, and Northern Mexico.

Prickly Pear is one of the most historical delicious fruits that posses a big number of health benefits, for example:

Diabetes:A mechanism of action remains to be discovered in diabetes; however, polysaccharides may be responsible for the plant's hypoglycemic activity.

Hyperlipidemidia

Two animal studies examined the effect of prickly pear seed oil on serum and lipid parameters in rats. An increase in high-density lipoprotein cholesterol (HDL) and a reduction in serum cholesterol was observed in rats treated with seed oil. Raw prickly pear had beneficial effects on hypercholesterolemia .

Inflammation

The mechanism of action is associated with the anti-inflammatory principle β-sitosterol.

Anti-inflammatory actions were demonstrated in Prickly Pears in an induced rat paw edema model. β-sitosterol from the fresh stems of prickly pear had potent anti-inflammatory activity in an adjuvant-induced chronic inflammation .

C-reactive protein and symptoms such as nausea, dry mouth, and anorexia were reduced in patients treated with prickly pear.

Ulcers

The prickly pear is famous for its excellent properties against ulcers.

Antioxidant

Prickly pear has an excellent antioxidant activity

Diuretic

Prickly pear fruit, and flower infusions increased diuretic properties in a rat model as well as humans.

Neuroprotective effects

Animal models in rats demonstrated that the flavonoids isolated from prickly pear had neuroprotective activity against oxidative injury induced in cortical cell cultures and neuronal damage induced by global ischemia.

Viral activity

Many studies reports antiviral action in animals and humans.

Wound healing

Histological evidence documents that topical application of polysaccharide extracts from prickly pear provided a good repair and healing of large, full-thickness wounds in a rat model.

Prickly Pear Fruit contains 220 ppm of **Shikimic Acid** the active ingredient of **Tamiflu!!**

The Most Effective Anti-Viral Anti-Flu Herbs:

Here is a list of the most effective anti-viral anti-flu used worldwide:

ANDROGRAPHIS PANICULATA:

The most effective anti-viral herb on earth. More details about its potential properties will be discussed in the following pages of this chapter.

AMLA FRUIT: Very rich in Vitamin C which is well known as an immunity enhancer and as anti-viral & anti-flu agent.

ANISE Tea: stimulates mucus secretion in lungs & throat.

BLACK SEED: very strong anti-bacterial, anti-bacterial, antibiotic, anti-microbial, anti-diabetic, anti-lipid, anti-cancerous and,anti-HIV and it increases immunity by 35% according to a clinical study published by the famous M.D. Ahmad Elkadi.To read more on the unique properties of black seed you can buy 2 books from **AMAZON.COM** discussing in details about 28 diseases treated by black seed!!!

CAMEL MILK: (See details below)

CATNIP Tea: relieves fever & digestive upset, relaxing effect.

CAYENNE: Added to fresh orange juice or soup to relieve congestion and increase mucus flow.

COCONUT OIL: Very strong anti-bacterial ,anti-bacterial, antibiotic,anti-microbial, anti-diabetic, anti-lipid, anti-cancerous,anti-HIV ,anti-pneumonia, anti-ashmatic and it increases immunity. The antiviral, antibacterial, and antifungal properties of the medium chain fatty acids/triglycerides (MCTs) found in coconut oil have been known to researchers since the 1960s. Research has shown that microorganisms that are inactivated include bacteria, yeast, fungi, and enveloped viruses. Much of this research is highlighted in the writings of Dr. Mary Enig .

ECHINACEA Immune stimulant that relieves major flu symptoms.

ELDERBERRY Prevents infections and shortens duration of flu.

ELECAMPANE: Expectorant. It relieves bronchial asthma , cold, flue ,and breathing difficulty .**More than 4000 asthmatics used it as a part of our herbal formula AZMA TECH TEA and all of them were cured from chronic and severe asthma!!!**

EPHEDRA Opens bronchial passages.

GARLIC Is an antibacterial and antibiotic that helps prevent infection. Eaten raw or taken in capsules.

GINGER A tea made by steeping the fresh, chopped root in boiling water for 20 minutes is used to soothe throat and ease congestion.

GREEN TEA: as a well-known anti-oxidant ,anti-bacterial and anti-viral.

HONEY & CINNAMON: Excellent combination for many symptoms including cold and flu.

HYSSOP: relieves mucus, cold and flu.

LEMON BALM: an excellent anti-viral agent and it is used extensively for herpes simplex viral infections I &II .It is a delicious tea with lemon flavor and taste and we tried it for most viral and bacterial infections.

MULLEIN Used as expectorant and to soothe sore throat.

NEEM LEAF EXTRACT: an excellent anti-viral, anti-bacterial ,anti-flu,anti-diabetic, anti-lipid,anti-cancerous and anti-HIV

OLIVE LEAF EXTRACT: an excellent anti-viral, anti-bacterial ,anti-flu,anti-diabetic, anti-lipid,anti-cancerous and anti-HIV

PROPOLIS: The most effective anti-biotic on earth and there are many studies show that proplis is equivalent to 132 antibiotic hence it is essential to be in the pockets of all family members!!.

Andrographis Paniculata Health Benefits

Andrographis is a herbal medicine derived from the Andrographis Paniculata shrub grown the moist, shady in India, China and throughout Southeast Asia. It is commonly referred to as 'Indian Echinacea' and is a popular Ayervedic and Chinese household remedy for the common cold, digestive issues, upper respiratory tract infections, flu and other sicknesses typified by fever. Although its use dates back easily a thousand years in these ancient medical traditions, there is a more recent historical reference to its potency. **In the Indian flu epidemic of 1919, the herb Andrographis is credited with the reversal of its**

onslaught. More recently, it popularity has spread to Scandinavia, where its dosages have been standardized and it has been widely recommended by doctors for two decades as a common remedy in treating these same winter ailments .

As research increases, so is our understanding of Andrographis' many activities and indications are that it may even play a role in cardiovascular and cancer treatments.

Andrographis Paniculata Benefits and Key Uses:

Colds, Flu & Sinusitis

Digestive problems

Cardiovascular

Anti-tumor

Clinical Applications

Andrographis and its various components have demonstrated a variety of effects in the body. Aspects stimulate the general immune activities, others inhibit the body's inflammatory mechanism and still others demonstrate not only anti-microbial abilities, but also are instrumental in killing certain tumor cells. Studies have also indicated that the active chemical, Andrographolide, helps to stop the clumping of blood platelets which is the clotting process that can lead to heart attacks .

How It Works?

For Colds, Flu and Sinusitis:

Andrographis compounds have shown very effective antivirus properties which appear to inhibit glycoprotein's in the virus. This impedes the viruses ability to invade cells in the body and replicate. It's andrographolide are currently being studied for the antiviral effects they have on avian bird flu virus, ebola virus and HIV .

It also has a major effect activating the general defense functions of the immune system by stimulating the production of antibodies as well as non-specific immune responses such as increased macrophage phagocytosis, rather than by any direct anti-microbial activity.

Clinical studies have demonstrated it's efficacy fighting colds, flu, sinusitis, familial mediterranean fever(FMF) and upper respiratory tract infections. It also has been demonstrated to reduce the risk of colds by 2.1 time and prevent flu and its complications.

Anti-inflammatory:

There appears to be a significant presence of flavanoids in the Andrographis Paniculata herb, which always have an anti-inflammatory affect. In vitro studies have shown that the flavinoid activities supressed the genetic expression of neutrofils, an inflammatory agent. Similarly, studies have indicated that a variety of inflammatory proteins, including COX-2, are reduced by the presence of Andrographoloid .

Anti-tumor :

In vitro andrographolide studies indicate an immuno-stimulating activity as well as a marked inhibitory effect. Its presence increases proliferation of lymphocytes and production of interleukin2, TNF-alpha production and cytotoxic activity of lymphocytes against certain cancer cell lines, as well as demonstrating potential direct anti-cancer activity by the induction of cell-cycle inhibitory protein p27 and decreased expression of cyclin-dependent kinase .

CAMEL MILK HEALTH BENEFITS:

Camel Milk the super food...

Camel milk, which is slightly saltier than traditional milk, is drunk widely across the Arab world and is well suited to cheese production.

It is is rich in **vitamins** B and C and has 10 times more iron than cow's milk.

Camel's milk is said to be an 'acquired taste', yet many people around the world depend on it. Its composition is closer to human milk than cow's milk is, so it is better for us. It also contains **antibodies, and these may help fight serious diseases like cancer, HIV/Aids, Alzheimer's and hepatitis B**. My patients used camel milk sucssesfully for liver cirrhosis, liver cancer, lung cancer,, eczema, psoriasis, asthma, pneumonia, cold and flu!!!It could be the 'super food' of the future in the West, and generate much-needed income for developing countries. The United Nations is calling for the milk to be sold to the West.

Will Camel milk become the 'Insulin' of the future?

Health benefits of camel milk are attributed to presence of high concentration of insulin-like protein and other factors that have a positive effect on the **immunity.** The fact that it does not coagulate easily in an acidic environment (e.g. in the stomach) makes it available for absorption in the **intestines**. The anti-diabetic action of camel milk has been attributed to the camel's choice (or is it default!) grazing/browsing on natural vegetation in the desert, including salty herbs and plants, some medicinal plants like the (neem).

In Somalia and Kenya , some diabetics who recognize the value of Camel milk are using Camel milk therapy to control their **Diabetes**.

Will Camel milk be the new Viagra?

Chapter *X*

Farmer Vimaram Jat, from the Indian state of Rajasthan who has fathered a child at the age of 88, put his virility down to **drinking** two to three liters of Camel milk a day. He has sexual intercourse every day and plans to do so until death!

Camel Milk based beauty products?

Camel milk is a natural source of Alpha-Hydroxy acids which are known to plump the skin and smoothe fine lines. Camel Milk soap provides a most luxurious bath experience. Our cosmetic creams which include camel milk showed amazing whitening and anti-wrinkele properties and women who used our creams became 20 years younger in face and skin(for more information visit our web sites:

(www.magicperfume.net and www.irisdeadsea.com)

Products from Camel milk are already hitting the shelves of shops such as soaps and yoghurts. An Austrian **chocolate** maker has joined forces with an Arabic Camel farm in Al-Ain (United Arab Emirates - UAE) to create a new delicacy - Camel milk chocolates. But as yet the chocolates are only available in the UAE but is deemed to conquer the world as the sweet ambassador of Arabia.

A French dairy company started to produce cheese, ice cream and other dairy products from camel milk!!!!

Will you give Camal Milk a try?

HIGH FEVER BEST HERBS:

1-Artemisia Annua(Wormwood):

Artemisia annua L. is an annual herb native of Asia, it has been used for many centuries for the treatment of fever and malaria and it is a well-known medicinal plant in Africa, and is still used effectively by people of many cultures. Uses range from treating cough, fever,flu, colic, headache, to intestinal parasites and malaria. In addition, Artemisia annua is frequently used as a moth repellent, and in organic insecticidal sprays.

2-Violet Tea:

One of the most effective herbs and flowers I used for more

Than 15 years for high fever which is the most dangerous symptoms of swine flu!!!

Essential Oils for Swine Flu:

Some essential oils used as few drops of eucalyptus and mint oils (part of our product **RELAX U**) can be very helpful to make a nice chest rub. Also can be used directly under nose to help clear nasal passages and ease breathing!!!!!

Frankincense essential oil: an excellent chest rub for cough, flu and inflammation.

Aromatherapy for Boosting Immunity

Basic Immune Tonic Blend:

3 drops lavender

3 drops lemon oil

2 drops eucalyptus

1 ounce carrier oil (almond oil)

Use as a body oil daily in the bath as part of a health-maintenance program, under nose and on chest for cold or flu.

Other herbs oils such as Echinacea, astragalus, goldenseal, bayberry, boneset, calendula, ginger, lemon balm, oregano, thyme, wild indigo and Oregon grape are also helpful.

SUMMARY OF THE PROTOCOL;

I know that I flood my reader with huge number of health secrets and he he/she may be confused how a shortcut healthy and effective program could be arranged.

For myself and my family I arranged the following program:

The best formula to protect myself from swine flu is a combination of:

Anti-viral herbs   with anti-flu herbs, anti-fever herbs and immunity boosting herbs in a form of herbal tea:

20% Mamey Leaf Powder

20% Andrographis Powder

10% Anise Powder

10% Licorice Powder

5% Lemon Balm Powder

10% Mint Dried Powder

5 % Black Seed Powder

10% Artemisia Powder

10% Violet Flower Powder

3 Cups of the above tea on daily basis , 2 cups of lemon mint tea, 2 table spoons of honey-cinnamon-propolis-baking powder mix.

If the above juice ingredients are not available we can use the following herbal tea:

20% anise powder

20% lemon balm

10% licorice

10% mint

10% black seed

10% hyssop

10% elderberry

10% violet flower

Combined with:

3 Cups of the above tea on daily basis , 2 cups of lemon mint juice, 2 table spoons of honey-cinnamon-propolis-baking powder mix.